Anti-Inflammatory Diet for Beginners:

Lose Weight and Reduce Inflammation, the Step by Step Guide to Heal the Immune System and Restore Overall Health.

Suzanne Miller

Contents

Introduction

What is Inflammation?

Inflammation is a diagnostic procedure with the biological purpose to start mending by expanding dissemination. It is a perplexing procedure including both the invulnerable framework and vascular framework and the interaction of different compound go-betweens. Expanded circulation brings white platelets and sustenance to the site of damage or contamination with the goal that attacking pathogens are murdered and harm might be fixed. Trademark indications of inflammation incorporate agony (dolor), heat (calor), swelling (tumor) and redness (rubor).

Inflammatory and non-inflammatory arthritis, these are the most widely recognized types of arthritis. What's the difference? Inflammatory arthritis is typically known as rheumatoid arthritis, where the non-inflammatory arthritis is best known as osteoarthritis. It is regularly the situation that a similar joint inflammation that causes arthritis may likewise be related to other medical issues. Inflammatory arthritis is an inflammatory illness condition coming about because of degeneration of cartilage in the joint, causing torment. Rheumatoid arthritis is an auto-save illness in which the body's invulnerable framework assaults joints, tissues, and organs. A diagnostic procedure which has a biological purpose of helping to recuperate by expanding the dissemination is known as inflammation. It is a procedure which includes the vascular framework and invulnerable framework. This additionally consists of the interaction of different synthetic arbiters and is known as an intricate procedure.

Here, the sustenance and the white platelets made by expanded flow to the spot of contamination or damage with the goal that the attacking pathogens being expelled and the harmed ones fixed. The qualities of inflammation are heat, redness, swelling, and agony. Inflammation is either treated by medications or the typical path by being on a specific eating routine. Prescriptions have very little to offer without reactions or the utilization of torment executioners, so characteristic mitigating nourishments been devoured for better execution with no hazard. In any case, different sustenances being processed differently, some of them advance inflammation while others expel it.

When Inflammation Goes Awry:

While some inflammation is useful and suitable for recuperating, chronic, or intemperate inflammation, filling no need produces harm. Chronic inflammation has awful notoriety because it is embroiled in different malady procedures, including (yet not constrained to) ...

- Immune system illnesses

- Joint inflammation

- Diabetes

- Alzheimer's illness

- Atherosclerosis (solidifying of veins that prompts heart assault and stroke)

- Add and adhd

- Sensitivities and asthma

- Malignant growths

- Fiery inside sickness

Delicate tissue swelling and synthetic go-betweens engaged with inflammation can likewise disturb nerve endings, adding to torment.

What is the Anti-Inflammatory Diet?

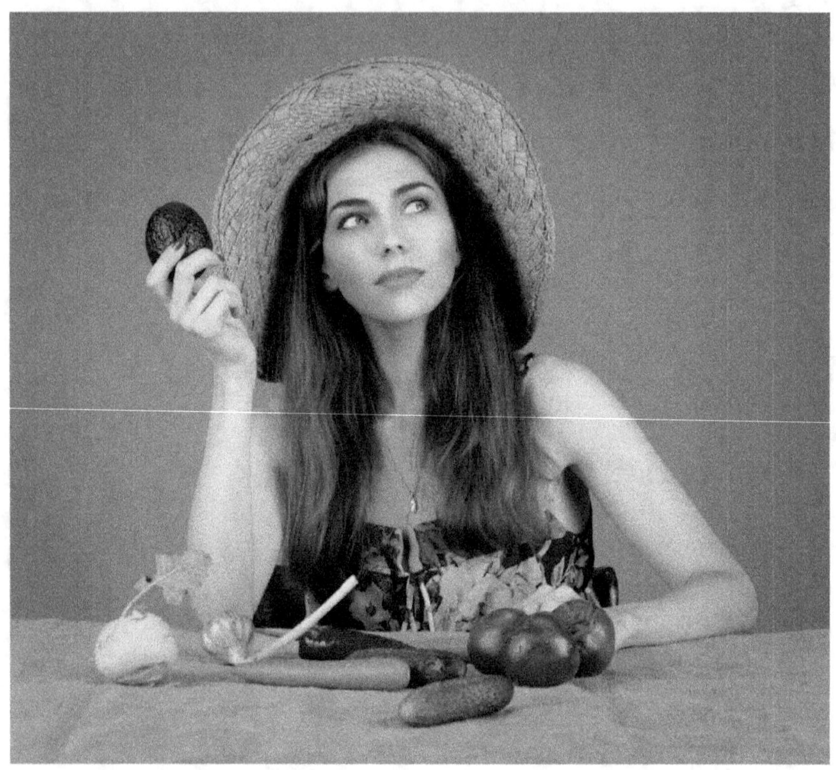

Different sustenances are processed; differently, some advancing inflammation and others diminishing it. The motivation behind the calming diet is to advance ideal wellbeing and mending by picking nourishments that decrease inflammation. If one can effectively control over the top inflammation through characteristic methods (like through diet), it lessens one's reliance on calming prescriptions that have undesirable and unfortunate reactions and don't take care of the fundamental issue. While mitigating prescriptions, (for example, NSAIDs) are a convenient solution to ease symptoms, they, at last, debilitate the resistant framework by harming the gastrointestinal tract which assumes a significant job in safe framework work.

Mitigating Diet Basics:

By and large, eat a bounty of new vegetables and organic products, entire grains, calming fats and nuts while constraining prepared nourishments, meat protein, milk items, refined sugars, artificial hues/flavors/sugars and sustenance sensitivities.

Vegetables:

Eat and Enjoy:

Appreciate a wealth of new vegetables and natural products in an assortment of hues (ideally natural). Products of the soil are loaded with nutrients, minerals, cell reinforcements, and fiber, which give the body the basic structure hinders for wellbeing. Models incorporate beans, squash, lintels, sweet potatoes, cruciferous vegetables, avocados, dull verdant greens... There are such vast numbers of decisions! Concerning organic products, pineapple and papaya are especially great because they are high in bromelain, a ground-breaking characteristic mitigating. Leafy foods additionally make extraordinary, solid bites.

Maintain a strategic distance from/Limit:

Maintain a strategic distance from produce that isn't developed naturally. Dangerous concoction buildups from herbicides and pesticides can remain and when ingested are outside aggravations to the framework. Numerous yields in North America are likewise hereditarily built and are put available without thorough scientific examination to decide security for human utilization. Independent research is, at last, being done to indicate the harmful impacts of devouring hereditarily modified life forms. Remote DNA is arbitrarily embedded into the genome of a yield. Models incorporate herbicide safe corn and soy, which are impervious to the herbicide Roundup, made by Monsanto. Generally, 90% of all corn and soy sold in North America is hereditarily modified. Likewise know about subsidiaries of hereditarily modified fixings, (for example, corn starch and corn syrup and so forth.). It has additionally been suggested that expending GMOs is a contributing component to the ascent insensitivities as the bodies are perceiving these nourishment substances as outside. By picking things with the "certified natural" name, you maintain a strategic distance from both GMOs and poisonous herbicides/pesticides.

For certain individuals, vegetables in the nightshade family may represent a worry. Instances of nightshade vegetables incorporate tomatoes, peppers, potatoes, and eggplant.

Nightshades contain alkaloids which are thought to exacerbate inflammation and joint harm in certain defenseless people with joint pain (however research is clashing). Along these lines, for certain people, restricting or dodging nightshade vegetables might be useful.

Fats:

Eat and Enjoy:

Appreciate sound, calming fats including olive oil, coconut oil, avocados, nuts, salmon and sardines. In people, there are two fundamental unsaturated fats, alpha-linolenic corrosive (an omega-3) and linoleic corrosive (an omega-6). These are "basic" because they are required for good wellbeing; however, the body does not blend them. Omega-3 fats are calming. Omega-6 fats can be genius fiery or mitigating (as it very well may be utilized by two different pathways). Researchers suggest that keeping the proportion of omega-6 to omega-3 somewhere in the range of 2:1 and 4:1 is best for wellbeing. The cutting edge diet will, in general, be high in omega-6 as it is copiously accessible in cooking oils. Subsequently, including rich wellsprings of omega-3 is significant, (for example, fish, flax and pecans particularly).

Evade/Limit:

Fats to restrict or keep away from incorporate margarine, spread, shortening, hydrogenated oils, trans fats, soaked fats, and milk fat. Omega-6 fats are extremely high in corn oil, safflower oil, and sunflower oil. Trans fats are connected with fiery maladies.

Meat:

Eat and Enjoy:

By and large, limit creature proteins because they will, in general, acidify the body and furthermore advance inflammation. When choosing creature protein, appreciate fish, poultry (particularly unfenced and naturally raised), sheep and omega-3 eggs.

Maintain a strategic distance from/Limit:

Cutoff meat, pork, shellfish, and processing plant cultivated eggs. All in all, grass-encouraged is better than grain-sustained. Maintain a strategic distance from burned sustenances, smoked nourishments, and cold cuts. Cold cuts contain nitrates and nitrites which advance malignant growth. Grilled nourishments contain sweet-smelling polycyclic hydrocarbons (PAHs) and heterocyclic amines (HCAs) which likewise advance cancerous growth.

Dairy:

Eat and Enjoy:

Appreciate dairy substitutes with some restraint, (for example, almond milk).

Maintain a strategic distance from/Limit:

Maintain a strategic distance from or limit dairy items by and large. This incorporates milk, yogurt, cheddar, and dessert. As we age, we lose the compound that overviews dairy, bringing about lactose prejudice and inflammation. The milk protein, casein, is likewise acidifying which (in spite of what numerous individuals are raised reasoning) burglarizes the bones of calcium.

Grains:

Eat and Enjoy:

Appreciate entire grains rather than refined grains. Refined grains will be grains in which the germ and wheat have been evacuated. This implies there is a loss of fiber, minerals, and nutrients. The great stuff is evacuated in return for a more drawn out period of usability. Some genuine instances of solid grains incorporate (natural) entire wheat/oats/bulgar/coucous, quinoa and whole oats (like steel-cut oats).

Entire grains are likewise a rich wellspring of complex starches. Complex starches (instead of essential sugars) will forestall spikes in your glucose level. Sugar advances inflammation.

Stay away from/Limit:

Stay away from our point of confinement refined starches, for example, white bread, baked goods, sweet things, and kinds of pasta.

Nuts:

Eat and Enjoy:

Appreciate nuts and nut margarines, for example, almonds, pecans, sesame seeds, pumpkin seeds, and flax.

Maintain a strategic distance from/Limit:

Maintain a strategic distance from a specific nut sensitivity.

Refreshments:

Eat and Enjoy:

Appreciate a lot of unadulterated, sifted water (staying away from chlorine, fluoride and different contaminants which are aggravations that advance inflammation). Other extraordinary decisions are lemon water and natural teas.

Stay away from/Limit:

Stay away from sugary soft drinks, organic product juice (with sugar included), and milk.

Flavors:

Eat and Enjoy:

Numerous flavors decrease inflammation. Some incredible models are turmeric, oregano, rosemary, ginger, garlic, and cinnamon. Bioflavonoids and polyphenols diminish inflammation and battle free radicals. Cayenne pepper is additionally calming, as it contains capsicum. Capsicum is regularly utilized in relief from discomfort creams.

Sugars:

Eat and Enjoy:

Appreciate stevia, molasses, maple syrup or nectar as better choices for refined sugar.

Keep away from/Limit:

Keep away from refined sugar, fructose and particularly high fructose corn syrup which advance inflammation. Evade artificial sugars.

Other:

Eat and Enjoy:

Appreciate aged nourishments, for example, kimchi, miso soup, and sauerkraut. Aged nourishments are probiotic and help to remake the invulnerable framework by supporting sound microflora in the gut and to diminish inflammation. Aged sustenances additionally will, in general, be anything but difficult to process and are likewise industrial facilities for B nutrients.

Stay away from/Limit:

When all is said in done, wipe out prepared sustenances, artificial hues, artificial flavors, and additives. Additionally, keep away from sustenances that you have a referred to affectability or allergy to as this advances inflammation. Second rate sensitivities are barely noticeable, so if you're uncertain, have a nourishment allergy test. The absolute most normal issue sustenances incorporate wheat (gluten), corn, soy, milk, and nuts.

All that we require for wellbeing can be found in nature. We need to pick well. If you need assistance and thoughts of what to eat, there are a lot of calming diet formula books accessible.

What Else Can You Do to Reduce Inflammation?

- Chiropractic care supports safe framework and diminishes inflammation!

- Reduce presentation to natural poisons, (for example, smoke)

- Reduce pressure

- Certain kinds of activity lessen inflammation - specifically, long haul, continuously dynamic preparing, staying away from over-effort.

Anti-inflammatory diet food list

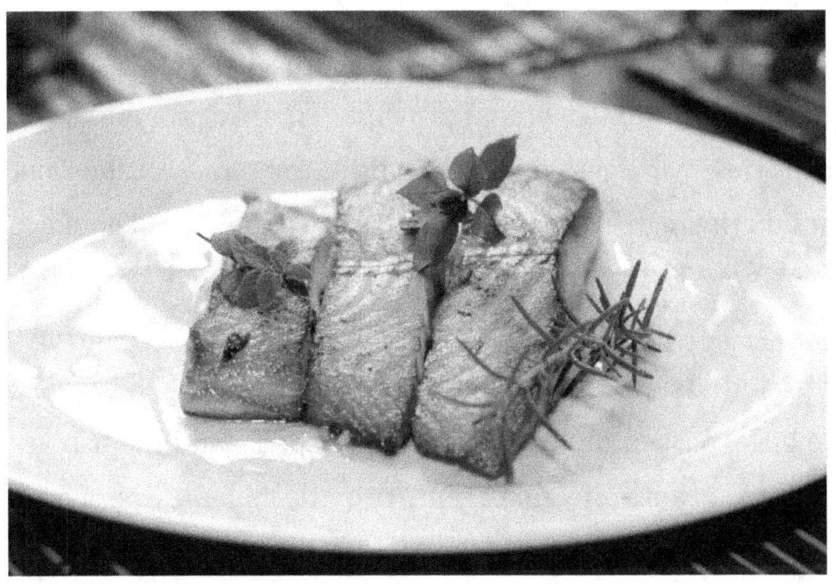

1 - Fish, mainly a virus water fish like salmon, trout, or fish, is stacked with mitigating omega-3 unsaturated fats. Numerous examinations affirm including fish (or fish oil) to one's eating routine will bring down aggravation.

Pick your fish cautiously There is much banter over wild fish versus ranch raised. Wild fish are typically higher in supplements and lower in fat than homestead built, because of their eating regimen and the activity they get swimming. Homestead raised fish, on the normal, have about 20% less protein and 20% more fat than wild got. Wild fish eat an eating regimen of little fish, shrimp, and red krill, which is the place the wealth of omega-3 EFAs in their substance starts.

They are likewise unfenced, and get copious exercise, decreasing their fat-content.

Ranch raised fish have sustained fishmeal pellets, typically made of ground, prepared and compacted mackerel, anchovies, sardines, and other little fish, which does not contain the high groupings of omega-3s than wild sustenance sources do. To impersonate the dark red shading that wild fish have, particularly salmon, most ranch-raised fish have bolstered a color alongside their feast. Because fish ranches are little, packed net walled in areas or pens, and the fish are encouraged anti-infection agents to battle maladies, parasites, and contaminations.

There have likewise been reports of high mercury content, both in wild and cultivated fish: the wild fish from living in sullied waters, and the cultivated fish from mercury tainting in their feed. Mercury in fish, for the most part, amasses in the skin, so don't eat the skin when eating any fish.

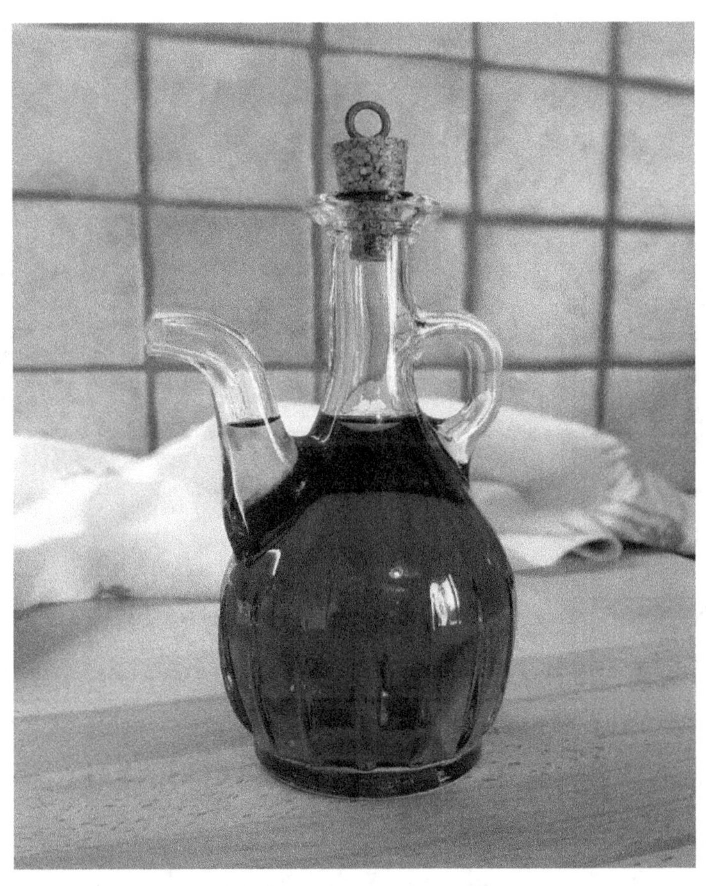

2 - Extra Virgin Olive Oil Olive oil is a rich wellspring of oleic corrosive; a mitigating oil. Olive oil likewise improves insulin work, subsequently bringing down glucose. Because of its low smoke point, olive oil isn't useful for profound singing. However, it is ideal for more beneficial cooking choices, for example, sauté and braising — Cook with olive oil rather than oils or shortening that are high in unfortunate trans-fats.

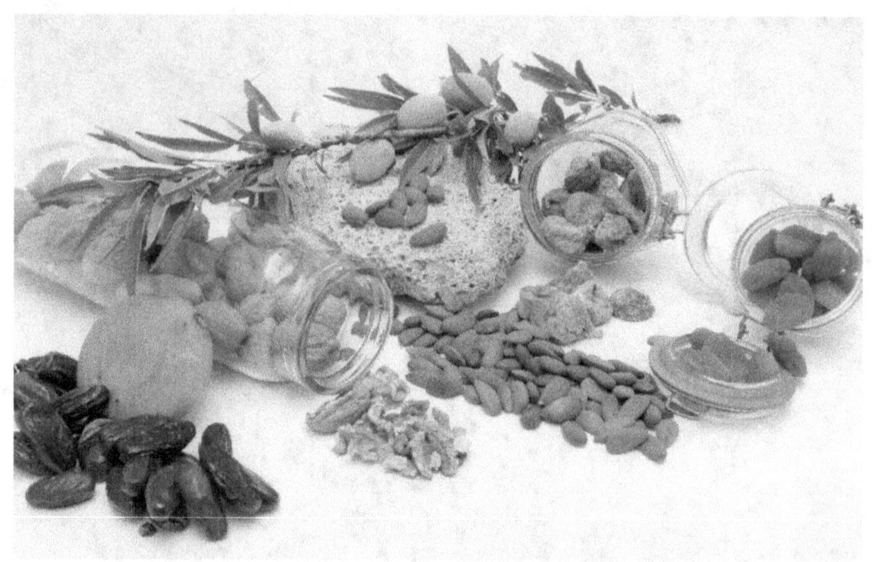

3 - Nuts Almonds, pecans, cashews, and different nuts are high in oleic corrosive, just as omega-3 unsaturated fats, fiber, protein, and other sound phytochemicals. Because a few nuts are high in fat, make sure to eat them with some restraint.

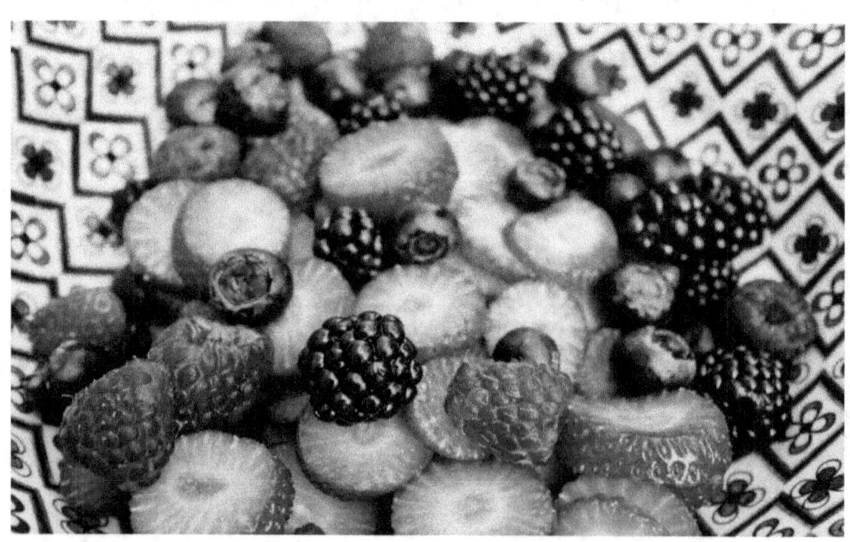

4 - Grapes Researchers report that grapes are high in flavonoids, which they accept have calming properties. As indicated by Medical news today "Now, researchers at the Johns Hopkins University School of Medicine have demonstrated that powdered grapes seem to diminish agony and aggravation in a rodent model of joint pain, where rodents' knees are excited utilizing a synthetic infusion." Perhaps drinking wine, as the Europeans know, can bring down irritation too.

5 - Cherries, particularly tart fruits, are a rich wellspring of antioxidants. Specifically, they contain a lot of anthocyanins, one of the most powerful enemies of oxidants, which give the fruits their rich, red shading. An investigation led by the Agricultural Research Service (ARS) researchers and their college partners proposes that fruits may lessen difficult joint irritation, just as diminishing the danger of other provocative conditions, for example, cardiovascular ailment and malignant growth.

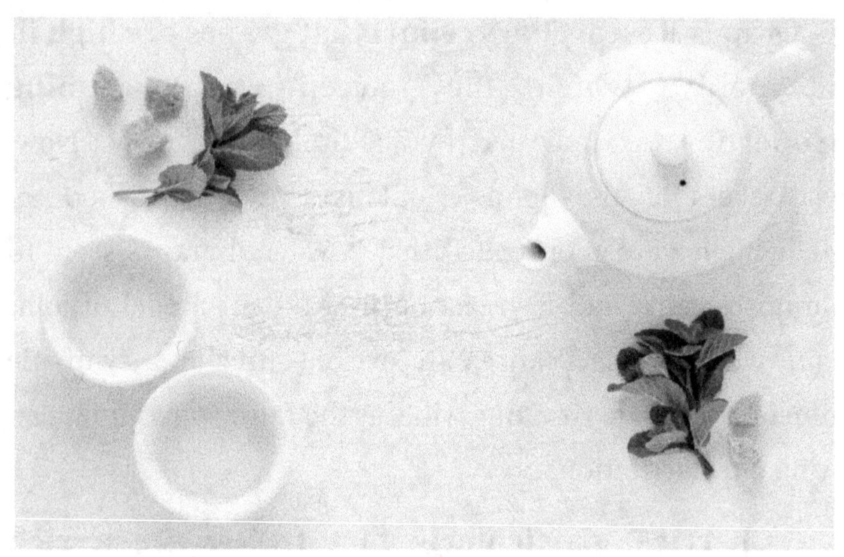

6 - Green Tea Green tea, which is unfermented, contains flavonoids called "catechins." Catechins are powerful antioxidants which are decimated during the handling and maturing process that different teas experience. Green tea contains about 27% catechins, instead of oolong (somewhat matured) which includes 23%, and dark tea (aged) which contains about 4%. Creature studies have demonstrated that green tea significantly diminished the seriousness of joint pain. As indicated by the National Center for Complementary and Alternative Medicine (NCCAM), green tea influences joint inflammation by causing changes in joint pain related insusceptible reactions.

If you find you have cerebral pains in the wake of devouring teas, you may have a hypersensitivity, the same number of individuals find. As usual, tune in to your body and see what works.

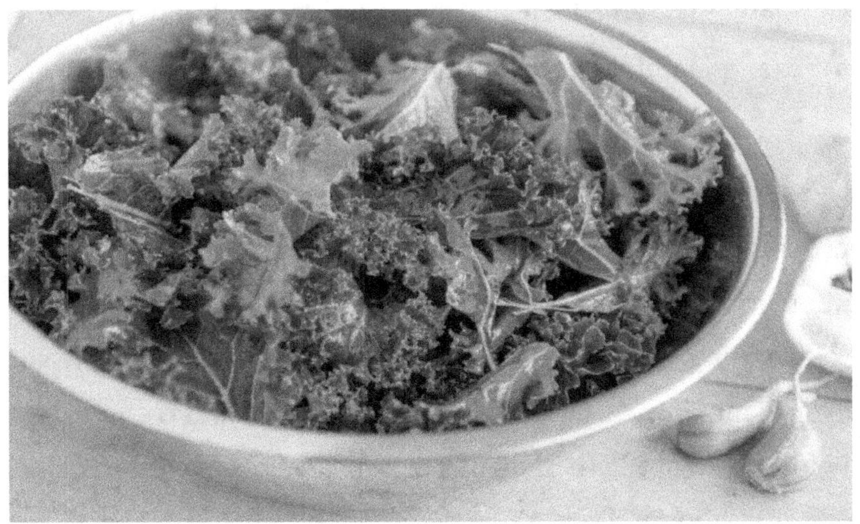

7 - Leafy Greens Green verdant vegetables, for example, spinach and kale, are stuffed with fiber, enemies of oxidants, and Omega 3s. Search for naturally developed produce, or make sure to wash altogether to expel the synthetics and pesticides that will result in general amass on the leaves.

8 - Broccoli A compound, 3,3'- diindolylmethane (DIM), found in broccoli and its kissing cousins, cauliflower and Brussel grows, has been appeared to battle irritation and help support the insusceptible framework. These super-veggies additionally contain sulforane, a phytonutrient that helps liver capacity and builds your body's common detoxification capacity. Eat them crude (solidified assortments of vegetables lose a great deal of nutritional worth) or steam them to protect the advantageous supplements, which can be separated by cooking strategies, for example, bubbling or broiling.

9 - Apples and red onions both contain quercetin, a compound that research has appeared to have calming properties, alongside different antioxidants. Most of the quercetin is in their skins, and it's what gives them their rich red shading, so don't strip apples before you eat them. Wash every single crisp food grown from the ground a long time before eating to help dispense with pesticides and composts.

10 - Water The newer, clean water you drink, the better. Your body is comprised of over 70% water, and continuous replenishment keeps poisons flushed from your framework, including joints, muscles, and blood.

As of late, with the expanded ubiquity of filtered water, there has been warmed discussion over faucet water versus filtered water. To choose which is better for you, you should realize what the differences are.

There is a dazing exhibit of decisions in filtered water accessible available today, from spring water, mineral water, well water, to shining water. While some of them originate from natural springs and other immaculate sources, over 25% of the filtered water sold originates from metropolitan sources.

Yes, you might drink faucet water!

Smart bundling messages have corralled the crowd attitude of an accommodating, idealistic open!

It's been dealt with, filtered and purified, at that point packaged and offered to you at a thousand-overlay increment in cost. There are no ebb and flow guidelines that power the bottler to the state where the water originates from, with the goal that unblemished mountain icy mass dissolves that you thought you were drinking may have in reality originated from a tap in Alaska or New Jersey.

Filtered water is no more advantageous than faucet water. Ebb and flow research recommend that it might be increasingly unsafe. BPA's, synthetic concoctions in the plastic of the containers themselves, can escape into the water you are drinking. (BPAs are known to cause neurological issues, in addition to other things.)

Notwithstanding the threats of the synthetic substances in the containers, there are other natural impressions to consider. Petroleum derivatives, with their related pollution and nursery gasses, are utilized to deliver the plastic containers. Transportation water contains far and wide uses progressively non-renewable energy sources, just as causing carbon pollution of air and conduits. While most plastic water jugs are recyclable, over 75% of them end up in landfills, or littering shorelines, lakes, and the sides of the street.

Take a gander at your faucet water.

Metropolitan water sources are thoroughly treated and tried by the EPA. EPA guidelines of contaminants are exacting, while the FDA guidelines for filtered water are a lot looser. Faucet water additionally contains fluoride, to help shield teeth from rot. In particular, the faucet water is very wallet cordial! Twenty ounces of water from the kitchen fixture costs pennies, yet twenty ounces of filtered water costs over $1.

If the flavor of the filtered water is the thing that keeps you getting it, consider adding a filter to your faucet water at home. There are numerous filters accessible in a colossal scope of costs, from essential pitchers that filter water for around $20, as far as possible up to complex frameworks for your whole house that cost a large number of dollars. Make sure to look at that it doesn't filter the fluoride that your teeth need. If you like the comfort of the versatile container, consider putting resources into a modest reusable jug made of a more secure, progressively tough plastic, for example, that used to ship water on a bike, or even a glass or metal bottle. Your condition and your wallet will value the exertion.

Certain Foods That Contribute to Inflammation

The rundown of foods to anticipate for that enemy of aggravation diet plan incorporates all wheat items, dairy things, potatoes, tomatoes, corn, sugar, citrus organic products, pork, business (nonorganic) eggs, shellfish, peanuts and nutty spread, espresso, liquor, juice, jazzed teas, pop, something containing hydrogenated oils, handled suppers, and browned foods.

Various of these suppers can lead straightforwardly to aggravation. For example, tomatoes and potatoes, which are component of the Salicaceae or nightshade group of vegetables, are perceived to cause aggravation. Tomatoes and potatoes should undoubtedly have stayed away from by anyone with joint inflammation of any sort. Dairy things merit referencing because they tend to turn out to be extremely higher in fat.

The measure of weight truly isn't the issue, even though, because the amount of fat-dissolvable harms which are put away inside the weight turns into the genuine issue. We realize that customarily raised dairy cows, and subsequently dairy items, are barraged with toxins as pesticide deposits on feed and genetically modified soy items in the feed.

Numerous cows, who are normally herbivores, are even sustained creature protein, which comprises of its own gathered poisons and consequently thus further builds the total poison load in dairy items. Like an outcome, dairy items add to the heap of poisons that the body's resistant program must technique and dispose of (or store if the body is under pressure and in this manner unfit to dispose of the toxins).

You may think about how you will get the calcium vital for bone wellbeing if you're approached to keep away from milk. Isn't maintaining a strategic distance from milk, especially unsafe for that advancement of youngsters' bones? The dairy business has made a sublime showing of showcasing the thought that everybody needs to drink milk to keep bones healthy and solid.

In truth, there are numerous nondairy wellsprings of calcium, including fortified soy, rice, oat, almond, and other nut milks. The whole body retains just around 30 percent from the calcium contained in dairy things. The Townsend Letter for Doctors and Individuals, inside an outline of over twenty different articles, presumed that sensitivity to dairy animals' milk is basic among grown-ups and kids.

Flawless milk proteins are perceived to invigorate the emission of proinflammatory cytokines in powerless people; for example, those with dairy animals' milk allergy. In expansion, just because, customary diet plan is to a great extent comprised of creature proteins, (for example, milk proteins), which are acidic, the whole body expels calcium from the unresolved issues balance the pH in the gastrointestinal framework. If one discovers they don't respond to dairy and wish to incorporate it in their diet, recommend is to eat just common dairy items.

They do exclude the pesticide deposits, hormones, and anti-microbial buildups typical dairy may incorporate. That is just because the bovines are held to higher nourishing guidelines and along these lines don't gather unnecessary harms through their diet. In any case, even natural dairy things shouldn't be devoured every day. The best-and an as often as possible disregarded substitute to drinking milk is drinking water.

somebody said he needs his patients to drink a large portion of their fat in liquid ounces of separated drinking water day by day. (one cup approaches eight liquid ounces. In this way, a single gauging 140 pounds should drink seventy liquid ounces of drinking water regularly, which works out to around nine cups, or a little more than two quarts.)

Drinking sifted water is significant essentially because it diminishes the poison load by sifting through undesirable metals, for instance, aluminum and lead, microorganisms, hormones, pesticide buildups, modern pollutants, solvents, lethal components, alongside other water-dissolvable poisons. Fluids to devour as a feature of the counter aggravation diet comprise of sifted drinking water and homegrown teas made with separated water.

All stimulated refreshments and drinks containing sugar are avoided. The juice is avoided just because it is extremely a major wellspring of concentrated sugar, even though it is a characteristic sugar. Inquire as to whether you can eat four oranges in a single sitting. If the appropriate response is no, at that point, you should not expend an eight-ounce glass of squeezed orange, which contains the identical measure of sugar yet comes up short on the helpful fiber content the entire natural product would have.

Liquor should be counteracted because it transforms into sugar once in the whole body. Espresso alongside other charged refreshments are saddling towards the liver because of their poison load and are exhausting towards the adrenal organs because of caffeine's effect on cortisol amounts. The adrenal organs, situated over the kidneys, are in charge of looking after vitality, creating sex hormones, adjusting pulse and glucose, and directing the pressure reaction.

If an individual's program is as of now troubled with physiological or mental stressors, caffeine will debilitate any pressure directing assets left inside the body. Caffeine additionally, detrimentally affects weight reduction and can cause tension, outrage, sleep deprivation, and irritability. Commercial eggs, meat, and pork are incorporated on the rundown of foods to stay away from to a great extent for precisely the same reasons that dairy is to progress toward becoming kept away from: just because of the poison content material and acidifying nature of the creature protein.

Pork and hamburger are higher in arachidonic corrosive, which advances aggravation. Some natural meat is permitted;

however, they should be eaten sparingly. Pork, even characteristic, isn't allowed on this diet plan because of its capability to animate an immune system reaction and because of its fat quality. Pigs have fundamentally the same as protein structures to people; consequently, expending pork can improve the opportunity of cross-responses inside the insusceptible program.

A cross-response happens when the invulnerable program responds towards the pork proteins which are so tantamount to human proteins, at the same time setting off a safe reaction against the body's very own cells.

Just because pigs frequently live in unclean conditions, have noncomplex assimilation, and will eat something, including their own young and considers them to have lower-quality fats, making them lower-quality sustenance. Studies have demonstrated that the obvious weight content in pork is genuinely elevated in arachidonic corrosive contrasted with hamburger, even though the genuine meat of the pig is lower in arachidonic corrosive. The calming diet is created to feed the whole body on all levels.

Pork isn't allowed on this diet plan for more than one reason: because of its abnormal amounts of arachidonic corrosive and because of its capability to make insusceptible framework irregularity. Common eggs which are free of hormone and pesticide deposits and that originate from unfenced chickens are allowed. However, they ought not to be eaten every single day because of their creature protein content.

Sugar causes various unusual responses inside the body and should be maintained a strategic distance from by all people. Sugar discourages the insusceptible program and doesn't give any supplements towards the diet plan. Drawn out high-sugar diets lead to higher glucose amounts, higher insulin levels, and elevated cholesterol amounts, all of which improve heart ailment hazard, insulin obstruction, and diabetes peril.

Shellfish and peanuts are kept away from as a feature of the counter aggravation diet essentially because numerous people have hypersensitivities to them. Peanuts additionally grow aflatoxin on their surface, which has been appeared to improve the occurrence of malignant growth in certain people; peanuts must be prepared cautiously to anticipate the generation of this substance. Corn is another normal allergen that should be stayed away from.

Ordinarily developed corn has regularly experienced a significant measure of genetic designing and been exposed to overwhelming assault with pesticides. Wheat merits talking about, basically because the customary diet plan has gone wheat insane. Should you need a decent point of view on wheat used in the present diet, ask any individual who has celiac sickness, that is an infection of gluten prejudice that outcomes in gut difficulties.

Accept from the ordinary American family and what they eat on a regular premise. As referenced over, one may have grain, toast, or flapjacks for breakfast, a sandwich for lunch, and afterward, pasta or pizza for supper. The average family may expend wheat multiple times ordinary. Today, wheat isn't what it was a hundred years back.

Wheat has been incredibly genetically modified; besides, numerous supplements are expelled inside the refining and handling of wheat. Genetically modifying wheat has raised its gluten content material to 90 percent, which is amazingly sporadic. It's conceivable that the genetic modification of wheat has changed its structure into something the whole body does not perceive as "sheltered to pass."

In their book Dangerous Grains, James Brady and Ron Hoggan depict gluten like a protein how the invulnerable framework responds to pathologically, creating irritation. Their hypothesis, upheld by proof, is that gluten annihilates healthy tissue by means of atomic mimicry, or cross-response. As indicated by an article distributed in the November 2001 issue from the diary Annals of Allergy, Asthma, and Immunology, the substances CRP and IL-6 are expanded during intense unfavorably susceptible responses.

Remember that CRP and IL-6 invigorate bothering. This same response can be seen with any nourishment hypersensitivity, wheat merely being a typical occurrence. Citrus natural products may improve bothering in the whole body; they likewise tend to irritate joint inflammation side effects. It isn't clear why citrus foods trigger provocative joint manifestations in specific individuals yet not others;

In various people with rheumatoid joint pain, one or significantly more from the foods to be maintained a strategic distance from on this diet plan will aggravate their condition. Once more, this does not imply that every one of these foods is fundamentally terrible for everyone. Much the same as a honey bee sting can trigger an extraordinary reaction in one individual and not in extra, and these suppers may trigger joint agonies in certain people; however, not others.

Remember that during the disposal and challenging period of the diet, you may start to expend these foods again to check whether you respond to them. For example, if you reintroduce peanuts and don't react negatively to them, you can expend them, however only one out of every odd day. (Keep in mind that one from the critical elements of a healthy diet is an assortment.)

Knowing your nourishment responses will be useful in treating and averting unending illness. Strangely, an individual may find that they respond to nonorganic corn, however not to natural corn. At long last, other than foods that normally trigger hypersensitivities or sensitivities, different dinners that should be maintained a strategic distance from are prepared suppers, dinners containing hydrogenated oils, and fricasseed foods. Foods containing hydrogenated oils, for example, fricasseed suppers, invigorate the discharge from the inflammation-promoting prostaglandins.

Any dinners that are prepared are probably going to incorporate vast amounts of additives, poisons, and colors, all of which contribute towards the body's overall harmful burden. Also, they have regularly been perched on racks for a considerable length of time or months before buy, unmistakably diminishing their degree of essential supplements.

Top Sources for the Anti-Inflammatory Diet

HEALTHY SWEETS

The amount: Sparingly

Healthy decisions: Unsweetened dried organic product, dim chocolate, natural product sorbet

Why: Dark chocolate furnishes polyphenols with cancer prevention agent movement. Pick dim chocolate within any event 70 percent unadulterated cacao and have an ounce a couple of times each week. Natural product sorbet is a superior choice than other solidified sweets.

RED WINE

The amount: Optional, close to 1 to 2 glasses for each day

Healthy decisions: Organic red wine

Why: Red wine has valuable cell reinforcement action. Limit admission to close to 1 to 2 servings for each day. If you don't drink liquor, don't begin.

SUPPLEMENTS

The amount: Daily

Healthy decisions: High-quality multivitamin/multimineral that incorporates vital cell reinforcements (nutrient C, nutrient E, blended carotenoids, and selenium); coenzyme

Q10; 2 to 3 grams of a molecularly refined fish oil; 2,000 IU of nutrient D3

Why: Supplements help fill holes in your diet when you can't get your day by day necessity of micronutrients.

TEA

How much: 2 to 4 cups for each day

Healthy decisions: White, green, oolong teas

Why: Tea is wealthy in catechins, cancer prevention agent intensifies that lessen aggravation. Buy fantastic tea and figure out how to blend it effectively for most extreme taste and medical advantages.

HEALTHY HERBS AND SPICES

The amount: Unlimited sums

Healthy decisions: Turmeric, curry powder (which contains turmeric), ginger and garlic (dried and new), bean stew peppers, basil, cinnamon, rosemary, thyme

Why: Use these herbs and flavors liberally to season foods. Turmeric and ginger are powerful natural calming agents.

Different SOURCES OF PROTEIN

How much: 1 to 2 servings per week (one segment is equivalent to 1 ounce of cheddar, one 8-ounce serving of dairy, one egg, or 3 ounces cooked poultry or skinless meat)

Healthy decisions: High-quality natural cheddar and yogurt, natural, omega-3 improved eggs, skinless poultry, grass-completed lean meats

Why: as a rule, attempt to decrease utilization of creature foods. If you eat chicken, pick natural, confine free chicken and expel the skin and related fat. Utilize natural dairy items respectably, basically yogurt and natural cheeses, for example, Emmental (Swiss), Jarlsberg, and genuine Parmesan. If you eat eggs, pick omega-3-improved eggs (from hens that are nourished a flax-dinner advanced diet) or natural eggs from unfenced chickens.

COOKED ASIAN MUSHROOMS

The amount: Unlimited sums

Healthy decisions: Shiitake, enokitake, maitake, shellfish mushrooms (and wild mushrooms if accessible)

Why: These mushrooms contain exacerbates that improve resistant capacity. Never eat mushrooms crude, and limit utilization of normal business catch mushrooms (counting cremini and Portobello).

Entire SOY FOODS

How much: 1 to 2 servings for every day (one serving is equivalent to ½ cup tofu or tempeh, 1 cup soy milk, ½ cup cooked edamame, or 1 ounce of soynuts)

Healthy decisions: Tofu, tempeh, edamame, soynuts, soymilk

Why: Soy foods contain is flavones that have cell reinforcement action and are defensive against malignancy. Pick whole soy foods over fractionated foods like detached soy-protein powders and impersonation meats made with soy confine.

FISH AND SHELLFISH

How much: 2 to 6 servings for each week (one serving is equivalent to 4 ounces of fish or seafood)

Healthy decisions: Wild Alaskan salmon (particularly sockeye), herring, sardines, and dark cod (sablefish)

Why: These fish are wealthy in omega-3 fats, which are emphatically mitigating. If you decide not to eat fish, take a molecularly refined fish-oil supplement that gives both EPA and DHA in a portion of 2 to 3 grams for every day.

HEALTHY FATS

How much: 5 to 7 servings for each day (one serving is equivalent to 1 teaspoon of oil, two pecans, one tablespoon of flaxseed, 1 ounce of avocado)

Healthy decisions: For cooking, utilize extra-virgin olive oil and expeller-squeezed grapeseed oil. Different wellsprings of healthy fats incorporate nuts (particularly pecans), avocados, and seeds, including hemp seeds and newly ground flaxseed. Omega-3 fats are additionally found in chilly water fish, omega-3 improved eggs, and whole soy foods. Natural, expeller-squeezed, high-oleic sunflower or safflower oils may likewise be utilized, just as pecan and hazelnut oils in servings of mixed greens and dim simmered sesame oil as a seasoning for soups and sautés.

Why: Healthy fats are those rich in either monounsaturated or omega-3 fats. Extra-virgin olive oil is rich in polyphenols with cell reinforcement movement.

Entire AND CRACKED GRAINS

How much: 3 to 5 servings per day (one serving is equivalent to about ½ cup of cooked grains)

Healthy decisions: Brown rice, basmati rice, wild rice, buckwheat groats, grain, quinoa, steel-cut oats

Why: Whole grains digest gradually, decreasing recurrence of spikes in glucose that advance irritation. Entire grains mean grains that are flawless or in a couple of enormous pieces, not entire wheat bread or different items produced using flour.

PASTA (AL DENTE)

How much: 2 to 3 servings for every week (one serving is equivalent to about ½ cup cooked pasta)

Healthy decisions: Organic pasta, rice noodles, bean-string noodles, and part entire wheat and buckwheat noodles like Japanese udo and soba

Why: Pasta cooked still somewhat firm (when it has "tooth" to it) has a lower glycemic record than completely cooked pasta. Low-glycemic-load sugars ought to be the main part of your starch admission to help limit spikes in blood glucose levels.

BEANS AND LEGUMES

How much: 1 to 2 servings for each day (one serving is equivalent to ½ cup of cooked beans or vegetables)

Healthy decisions: Beans like Anasazi, adzuki and dark, just as chickpeas, dark looked at peas, and lentils

Why: Beans are rich in folic corrosive, magnesium, potassium, and solvent fiber. They are a low-glycemic-load food. Eat them very much cooked either entire or pureed into spreads like hummus.

VEGETABLES

How much: 4 to 5 servings for every day least (one serving is equivalent to 2 cups plate of mixed greens or ½ cup vegetables cooked, crude, or squeezed)

Healthy decisions: Lightly cooked dim verdant greens (spinach, collard greens, kale, Swiss chard), cruciferous vegetables (broccoli, cabbage, Brussels grows, kale, book choy, and cauliflower), carrots, beets, onions, peas, squashes, ocean vegetables and washed crude serving of mixed greens

Why: Vegetables are wealthy in flavonoids and carotenoids with both cancer prevention agent and mitigating action. Go for a broad scope of hues, eat them both crude and cooked, and pick natural when conceivable.

Natural products

How much: 3 to 4 servings for each day (one serving is equivalent to 1 medium-size bit of organic product, ½ cup hacked natural product, ½ cup of a dried natural product)

Healthy decisions: Raspberries, blueberries, strawberries, peaches, nectarines, oranges, pink grapefruit, red grapes, plums, pomegranates, blackberries, fruits, apples, and pears – all lower in glycemic load than most tropical organic products

Why: Fruits are wealthy in flavonoids and carotenoids with both cell reinforcement and mitigating movement. Go for a wide scope of hues, pick a natural product that is new in season or solidified, and purchase natural when conceivable.

WATER

The amount: Throughout the day

Healthy decisions: Drink unadulterated water or beverages that are for the most part water (tea, exceptionally weakened natural product juice, shimmering water with lemon) for the day.

Why: Water is essential for generally speaking working of the body.

The Food Pyramid

The Food Pyramid is intended to make healthy eating simpler. Healthy eating is tied in with getting the right measure of supplements – protein, fat, sugars, nutrients, and minerals you have to keep up great wellbeing.

Foods that contain a similar kind of supplements are assembled on each of the racks of the Food Pyramid. This gives you a decision about different foods from which to pick a healthy diet. Following the Food Pyramid as a guide will enable you to get the correct equalization of nutritious foods inside your calorie goes. Studies demonstrate that we take in an excessive number of calories from foods and savors high fat, sugar, and salt, on the first-rate of the Food Pyramid. They give almost no of the essential nutrients and minerals your body needs. Restricting these is fundamental for healthy eating.

So more or less, healthy eating includes:

a lot of vegetables, a plate of mixed greens and natural product

a serving of whole meal grains and pieces of bread, potatoes, pasta, and rice at each supper - go for wholegrain assortments at every possible opportunity

some milk, yogurt, and cheddar

some meat, poultry, fish, eggs, beans, and nuts

a minimal quantity of fats, spreads, and oils

what's more, a minimal quantity or no foods and savors high fat, sugar, and salt

Supplements

If you eat a shifted and adjusted diet, at that point there is typically no compelling reason to take any food supplements – you'll get all that you need from your food. The one particular case to this is folic corrosive. All ladies of kid bearing age who could end up pregnant should take a supplement of 400µg (micrograms) folic corrosive every day. If a lady becomes pregnant, she should keep on taking the supplement during the initial twelve weeks of pregnancy.

The Healthy Eating Food Pyramid

Adjusted eating regimen is a key to remain healthy. Pursue the "Healthy Eating Food Pyramid" control as you pick your food. Grains ought to be taken as a significant dietary source. Eat more foods grown from the ground. Have a reasonable measure of meat, fish, egg, milk, and their choices. Diminish salt, fat/oil, and sugar. Cut back excess from meat before cooking. Pick low-fat cooking techniques, for example, steaming, stewing, stewing, bubbling, singing or cooking with non-stick broiling skillet. Likewise, lessen the utilization of broiling and profound fricasseeing. These can enable us to accomplish adjusted eating routine and advance wellbeing.

What amount of different sorts of food would it be a good idea for you to eat to remain healthy?

Eat the Right Food

Since different foods have different health benefits, it is beyond the realm of imagination to expect to get every one of the supplements we need from a solitary food. As indicated by the Healthy Eating Food Pyramid, we need to eat an assortment of foods among all food bunches just as inside each gathering to get different supplements and meet day by day needs.

Eat the Right Amount

Neither eating an excess of nor too little is useful for the wellbeing. Consistently, we need a specific measure of supplements to keep up ideal wellbeing. If we don't eat enough, under-nourishment and symptoms of lack are probably going to create; while over-sustenance and heftiness can become about when we devour an inordinate measure of food. Subsequently, we need to eat an appropriate standard of food to remain healthy.

Healthy Eating Food Pyramid

Eat Most - Grains

Eat More - Vegetables and organic products.

Eat Moderately - Meat, fish, egg, and options (counting dry beans) and milk and choices.

Eat Less - Fat/oil, salt, and sugar.

Drink adequate measure of liquid (counting water, tea, clear soup, and so on) consistently.

Healthy Eating Food Pyramid for Children (matured 2 to 5)

Grains: 1.5 - 3 dishes

Vegetables: in any event 1.5 servings

Natural products: at any rate one serving

Meat, fish, egg, and choices: 1.5 - 3 tales

Milk and choices: 2 servings

Fat/oil, salt, and sugar: eat the least.

Liquid: 4 - 5 glasses

Healthy Eating Food Pyramid for Children (matured 6 to 11)

Grains: 3 - 4 dishes

Vegetables: in any event two servings

Natural products: at any rate two servings

Meat, fish, egg, and choices: 3 - 5 taels

Milk and choices: 2 servings

Fat/oil, salt, and sugar: eat the least

Liquid: 6 - 8 glasses

Healthy Eating Food Pyramid for Teenagers (matured 12 to 17)

Grains: 4 - 6 dishes

Vegetables: in any event three servings

Natural products: in any event two servings

Meat, fish, egg, and choices: 4 - 6 taels

Milk and choices: 2 servings

Fat/oil, salt, and sugar: eat the least.

Liquid: 6 - 8 glasses

Healthy Eating Food Pyramid for Adults

Grains: 3 - 8 dishes

Vegetables: at any rate three servings

Organic products: at any rate two servings

Meat, fish, egg, and options: 5 - 8 taels

Milk and options: 1 - 2 servings

Fat/oil, salt, and sugar: eat the least.

Liquid: 6 - 8 glasses

Healthy Eating Food Pyramid for Elderly

Grains: 3 - 5 dishes

Vegetables: at any rate three servings

Organic products: at any rate two servings

Meat, fish, egg, and options: 5 - 6 taels

Milk and options: 1 - 2 servings

Fat/oil, salt, and sugar: eat the least.

Liquid: 6 - 8 glasses

Comments

One tael is identical to around 40 grams (crude meat).

The above proposals are expected for healthy people as they were. Those with chronic diseases and specific wholesome needs ought to counsel their family specialists and dietitians for individualized dietary suggestions.

Food Exchange List:

One bowl of grains is equal to:

Cooked rice, one bowl

Cooked noodles, 1¼ dishes

Bread, two cuts

One serving of vegetables is equal to:

Cooked vegetables, ½ bowl

Crude vegetables, one bowl

One serving of the natural product is identical to:

Medium-sized apple, one-piece

Kiwi, two pieces

Natural product cuts, ½ bowl

One tael of meat is equal to:

Cooked meat, 4-5 cuts

Egg, one-piece

Luxurious tofu, one-piece

One serving of milk and choices is identical to:

Low-fat milk, 1 cup (240ml)

Low-fat cheddar, two cuts

Low-fat plain yogurt, one-pot (150ml)

Significance of Food Pyramids

Gives Dietary Guidance

The essential advantage of food pyramids is that they give dietary direction in a simple to-pursue visual arrangement. In 2011, the USDA supplanted its pyramid with a vivid four-segment plate with a cup as an afterthought called MyPlate. It fills in as a less complex manner to speak to healthy eating designs. The thought is as yet the equivalent, to represent the five food gatherings - organic products, vegetables, grains, protein, and dairy - as a way to enable you to assemble healthy, well-adjusted suppers.

Improves Eating Habits

Numerous individuals need to eat more beneficial; however, don't have the foggiest idea where to begin. Food pyramids and plates give direction on what foods to eat a greater amount of and which foods to decrease. My Plate urges you to eat more products of the soil, as the food symbol is isolated into four fundamental areas, with one quarter for leafy foods quarter for vegetables. Most Americans neglect to get enough products of the soil, so filling a large portion of your plate with them is a decent spot to begin.

Goes about as a Reminder

Food symbols help you to remain on track in getting the suggested day by day prerequisites. Print out MyPlate and post it or another food symbol on your cooler, in your office or in a spot where you'll see it consistently. It bumps you to eat invigoratingly and helps you to remember which foods you've just eaten and which ones you have to incorporate into your next dinner. For instance, if your morning meal for the day rejected dairy, MyPlate reminds you to have a tidbit like a yogurt or to incorporate low-fat dairy with lunch.

Utilizing Food Icon Guides

The USDA MyPlate is anything but difficult to pursue. The objective is to fill a large portion of your plate with foods grown from the ground, a quarter with protein and the other quarter with grains; the cup reminds you to have a serving of dairy. Employees at the Harvard School of Public Health constructed the Healthy Eating Pyramid and Healthy Eating plate as options in contrast to the USDA's MyPlate. The HSPH food symbols give nitty-gritty direction progressively. Its segments remind you likewise to have nuts, seeds, and beans; pick entire grains; eat two week after week servings of fish; expend healthy oils; diminish red meat; limit sugary beverages, desserts, salt and refined grains; participate in normal exercise; and devour liquor with some restraint if you drink.

Revealing Nature's Best Anti-Inflammatory Herbs For Control Of Chronic Inflammation

Chronic inflammation is the key driver of an enormous number of chronic diseases, including coronary illness, diabetes, joint pain, psoriasis, and Alzheimer's disease. Even though there is a massive determination of mitigating drugs, the requirement for more secure calming treatment is kept on expanding because of well-perceived unwanted effects identified with prolonged haul utilization of mitigating drugs. Moreover, there is a rising wellbeing concern to tranquilize medicate cooperation.

The old Chinese and Ayurveda medicine offer an elective answer for inflammation help. Numerous restorative plants utilized in Traditional Chinese Medicine and Ayurvedic Medicine for a great many years have mitigating properties. In light of long stretches of research on inflammation-related diseases and calming drugs and herbs, they locate that mitigating herbs are overlooked and underutilized in doing combating chronic inflammatory sicknesses.

To create protected and important mitigating items for neglected wellbeing needs, they dedicate quite a while to look for best calming herbs that could convey safe inflammation alleviation for different wellbeing conditions. It is accepted that the decision of nature's best mitigating herbs ought to be founded on:

- Long and extraordinary viability records from conventional medicine

- Abundant pharmacological investigations distributed in therapeutic diaries

- Solid proof from clinical investigations utilizing propelled instruments of current medicine

- Well-settled wellbeing records

The accompanying herbs have been included the rundown of Nature's Best Anti-inflammatory Herbs:

Ground-breaking Anti-Inflammatory Herb - Scute

Scute (Scutellaria baicalensis, Huang qin) has been utilized for a considerable length of time in customary medicine to treat inflammation, contaminations, sensitivities, disease, and cerebral pains. It has been comprehensively inquired about in modern-day medicine with over 1200 articles referenced in PubMed.

Scute has been appeared to have calming, hostile to bacterial, antifungal, against viral, unfriendly to unfavorably susceptible, and hostile to tumor properties. It is one of the most usually utilized Chinese herbal medicine in Eastern and Western medicines.

The bioactivity of this herbal medicine is because of the extraordinary rummaging exercises of the flavone segments. The principle dynamic fixings bringing down inflammation incorporate baicalein, baicalin, and wogonin.

In light of distributed scientific and clinical research, Scute and its dynamic fixings

- Inhibit a wide scope of proinflammatory arbiters including cyclooxygenase-2, leukotriene B4, IL-1 beta, IL-2, IL-6, IL-12, TNF-alpha, 12-lipoxygenase and prostaglandin E2.

- Reduce the creation of nitric oxide and free radicals. So far, more than 60 flavonoids have been found in the foundation of Scute.

- Suppress disease cell development and prompt passing of malignant growth cells. New outcomes demonstrated that flavone parts of Scute are poisonous to tumor cells, however non-dangerous to ordinary cells.

- Diminish diabetic oxidative pressure, the underlying driver of full diabetic scale and miniaturized scale vascular intricacies. When joined with hostile to diabetic drugs, Scute raises liver cancer prevention agent compounds, helps insulin levels, and reduces triglycerides and cholesterol levels.

- Protect DNA from harmful changes, invigorate fix of harmed DNA.

- Inhibit type I and II touchiness responses in asthma and hypersensitivities. Ongoing screening of more than 2000 plants, Scute has been identified as one of the main two herbs that indicated most dominant enemy of histamine effects.

- Protect nerve cells from damage and harm through a few ways, i.e., initiating qualities that control synapse survival, expanding cerebral blood move through angiogenesis and neurogenesis, lessening neurotoxic components and master inflammatory operators delivered in mind because of ordinary and strange cerebrum maturing.

- Display an expansive range of hostile to viral and against HIV exercises.

- Block invasion of invulnerable cells and reduce inflammatory responses that are associated with atopic dermatitis/skin inflammation.

- Suppress UVB-incited MMP-9 and VEGF, the causal variables of skin aggravation and harm.

Age-old Anti-inflammatory Herb - Coptis

Coptis has been archived as one of the most established Chinese medicine. Coptis is perhaps the most grounded herb to take out warmth, dry sogginess, and poisons.

Coptis has been utilized as a principle element for treating inflammatory conditions, for example, intestinal and lung contaminations. It is additionally one of the essential fixings in skin solutions for psoriasis, dermatitis, skin break out, canker, and neurodermatitis.

Coptis has been widely examined in current medicine with more than 2600 articles distributed in PubMed. Pharmacological effects of Coptis comprise of an expansive range of antibacterial, hostile to contagious, against viral, and anti-inflammatory exercises. Other than its calming properties, it is likewise a vasodilator and has unfriendly to pyretic, against looseness of the bowels, against ulcer, and hostile to tumor effects.

In light of scientific and clinical examinations, Coptis and its dynamic fixings

- Inhibit inexhaustible inflammatory middle people and cell surface atoms associated with inflammatory responses.

- Enhance insulin affectability, increment articulation of insulin receptors, lower glucose, and reduce insulin opposition and type 2 diabetes.

- Reduce arrangement of free radicals and oxidative pressure, avert oxidative harm, and radiation-prompted damage.

- Suppress neuroinflammatory responses, give defensive impact in different neurodegenerative and neuropsychiatric issue, for example, Alzheimer's disease, cerebral ischemia, mental melancholy, schizophrenia, and tension.

- Exhibit against the proliferation and hostile to malignancy movement through different systems.

- Prevent glucocorticoid-initiated bone misfortune by restraining bone resorption and improving bone development.

- Induce apoptosis of hyper-dynamic invulnerable cells, subdue auto-resistant responses.

- Suppress development of fat cells, anticipate heftiness, and against insane medication initiated weight gain.

Astonishing Anti-inflammatory Herb Tumeric

Turmeric (Curcuma longa) has been utilized in Ayurvedic medicine and conventional Chinese medicine for a considerable length of time. It is generally used in traditional medicine to treat the biliary issue, anorexia, hack, diabetic injuries, hepatic issue, stiffness, and sinusitis. The dynamic segment of Turmeric is curcumin, which manages various targets, including translation factors, development factors, cell cycle proteins, inflammatory cytokines, chemicals, and cell surface bond particles.

Turmeric has gotten impressive enthusiasm as a potential helpful operator for the counteractive action and treatment of different dangerous diseases, joint pain, sensitivities, Alzheimer's disease, and other inflammatory ailments.

Because of scientific and clinical examinations, turmeric and its dynamic fixing curcumin

- Induce cell cancer prevention agent barriers and shield cells from oxidant challenge and maturing.

- Shield neurons and reduce neuron misfortune, improve learning and memory shortfalls by ensuring the sensory system against oxidative pressure.

- Prevent seizures and ensure against seizure prompted memory weakness.

- Improve insulin affectability and reduce glucose levels.

- Slow down the corruption of joint ligament and advance chondrocyte digestion in osteoarthritis.

- Diminish malignant growth cell development and metastasis in lung disease, prostate malignancy, bosom malignancy, and cancerous colon growth.

- Enhance twisted recuperating by expanding collagen creation and improving tissue structure and capacity.

- Protect skin from UV harm by hindering network debasing chemicals, key controllers of collagen debasement and photo aging.

- Prevent chronic bright B (UVB)- illuminated skin harm incorporating changes in skin thickness and versatility, pigmentation, and wrinkling.

Curcumin has low water solvency and poor assimilation through the digestive system. To beat these constraints, an enormous sum or detailing with different fixings is proposed.

Inflammatory Bowel Disease

The noninfectious inflammatory intestinal disease is recognized from irresistible elements by rejection: repetitive scenes of mucopurulent (i.e., containing bodily fluid and white cells) bleeding looseness of the bowels described by the absence of good societies for irresistible creatures and inability to react to anti-infection agents alone.

Just because intensifications and abatements portray inflammatory bowel sickness, proper responses to treatment are difficult to recognize from unconstrained reductions happening as part of the natural foundation of the disease. The trigger of noninfectious inflammatory intestinal disease is obscure disregarding advancement in knowing its pathogenesis.

There are two types of chronic inflammatory bowel disease: Crohn's disease, which is transmural and granulomatous in character, happening anyplace along the GI tract, and ulcerative colitis, which is shallow and confined towards the colonic mucosa. The reasons for an inflammatory intestinal ailment are obscure regardless of advancement in understanding its pathogenesis.

A blend of hereditary possibility and ecological variables are recognized as significant components in the pathogenesis of the inflammatory intestinal disease. A blast of recently recognized vulnerability qualities for every Crohn's disease and ulcerative colitis are now found through genome-wide affiliations.

These investigations assessed a large number of single nucleotide polymorphisms (SNPs) in a massive amount of sufferers with inflammatory intestinal ailment and contrasted them with individuals without having the disease. These examinations have discovered that various gatherings of vulnerability qualities that comprise of modulators of insusceptible capacity and cooperation with microorganisms.

Numerous environmental factors are already speculated to lead to the improvement of Crohn's disease, such as microorganisms (bacteria and viruses), nutritional elements, genetic elements, defective immune responses, and psychosocial elements. The normal gut can modulate frank inflammatory responses to its constant bombardment with dietary and microbial antigens within the lumen.

This modulation might be defective in Crohn's illness, resulting in uncontrolled inflammation. There has been considerable interest in the role of cytokines, this kind of as interleukins and tumor necrosis aspect, in Crohn's disease. Cytokine profiles of TH1 and TH17 groups have been implicated in Crohn's illness.

Mice lacking the TH1-inhibiting cytokine interleukin-10 have a TH1 cytokine profile and produce a Crohn's disease-like irritation of the intestine. Monoclonal antibodies to tumor necrosis aspect (TNF) reduce inflammation in these animals and patients.

Similar elements might lead towards the pathogenesis of ulcerative colitis, such as infections, allergies to dietary components, immune responses to bacteria and self-antigens, and psychosocial elements. In mice, targeted disruption of the genes for that T-cell receptor and also the cytokine IL-2 results in GI tract illness resembling ulcerative colitis.

The two kinds of inflammatory bowel ailment have highlight differences and in numerous examples, significant cover in the way of introduction. The highlights essential to all types of inflammatory intestinal disease are mucosal ulceration and inflammation from the GI tract, undefined, truth be told, from that which can happen intensely during intrusive irresistible loose bowels.

Different factors other than the nearness of significant-quality things, for example, irresistible specialists, modified host safe responses, resistant interceded intestinal harm, psychologic components, and wholesome and ecological components, may add to a last regular pathway of disarranged insusceptible reaction.

Clinical Manifestations:

1) Crohn's Illness: Crohn's disease, most, as a rule, happens in the distal ileum. In any case, the circulation of the disease may likewise include the colon or less normally some other locale from the GI tract, (for example, the oral hole, throat, stomach, and proximal small digestive system).

A trademark highlight is that spots of ulceration and inflammation happen in a broken manner and incorporate the entire thickness from the intestinal divider. A repeat of the disease can occur in beforehand uninvolved locales of the digestive system and can even include adjoining mesentery and lymph hubs.

The blend of profound mucosal ulceration and submucosal thickening gives the included mucosa a trademark "cobblestone" look. Aperture, fistula development, sore arrangement, and minimal intestinal deterrent are successive issues of Crohn's disease, albeit an inactive course occurs in many sufferers. The full-thickness contribution from the intestinal divider may incline to these entanglements.

Frank seeping from the mucosal ulcerations can be either treacherous or huge, as can protein-losing enteropathy. Another fundamental complexity is a conceivable expanded frequency of intestinal malignancy. Sufferers with Crohn's disease regularly manifest manifestations outside of the GI tract.

Most for the most part, inflammatory disarranges from the joints (joint inflammation), skin (erythema nodosum), eye (uveitis, iritis), mucous films (aphthous ulcers of the buccal mucosa) bile conduits (sclerosing cholangitis), and liver (immune system chronic vigorous hepatitis) are likewise seen in these sufferers. The renal issue, especially nephrolithiasis, is seen in a solitary third of patients with Crohn's disease, most likely identified with expanded oxalate assimilation related to steatorrhea.

Amyloidosis is extremely a genuine intricacy of Crohn's disease, as is thromboembolic sickness. Every one of these entanglements is presumably impressions of the foundational character of the inflammatory technique. Sufferers are habitually malnourished and show proof of supplement inadequacy states.

2) Ulcerative Colitis: as opposed to Crohn's ailment, bothering in Ulcerative Colitis is limited to the mucosa from the colon and rectum. It ordinarily starts at the anorectal intersection and broadens proximally. At a single time, it was accepted that ulcerative Colitis and Crohn's disease had been particular elements.

This view depended on the perception of trademark necrotic sores from the colonic sepulchers of Lieberkuhn, named "grave abscesses" in sufferers with ulcerative Colitis. In any case, it's currently perceived that in 10% of patients, locales normal for both Crohn's sickness and ulcerative Colitis are available.

The diseases are tantamount in the introduction (e.g., ridiculous looseness of the bowels and malabsorption) and in probably a portion of the entanglements (e.g., protein-losing enteropathy and unhealthiness), reflecting across the board contribution from the mucosa in the two elements.

All things considered, because ulcerative Colitis, for the most part, is confined to the mucosa, impediment, puncturing, and fistula arrangement aren't standard intricacies. Most sufferers have a mellow disease, and, similarly, as with Crohn's sickness, a few sufferers will have just a solitary or two scenes all through their lifetimes.

For new reasons, the shot of carcinoma appears to be considerably more prominent in ulcerative Colitis than in Crohn's disease. Harmful megacolon might be the solitary entanglement of ulcerative Colitis that conveys a high possibility of aperture. Its motivation is new. Both ulcerative colitis and Crohn's disease can go into abatement after treatment with first-line mitigating specialists, for example, sulfasalazine and glucocorticoids.

Crohn's ailment additionally reacts to treatment that uses monoclonal antibodies against the inflammatory cytokine, TNF. These antibodies tie to and repress this cytokine. Of late, treatment with against TNF monoclonal antibodies might be used in patients with ulcerative colitis as well. Because of potential intricacy of genuine, even life-compromising contamination, these drugs are used distinctly of severe examples.

The characteristic foundation of the two diseases is of times of abatement hindered by vivacious disease; restorative treatment all through intensifications are coordinated toward active measures and endeavors at initiating reduction. Because these ailments can repeat directly after resection of included areas of the GI tract, employable administration is generally confined to help of life-undermining intestinal deterrent or to die.

Because of the variable reaction rate and furthermore the great danger of side results, treatment with immunosuppressive operators this sort of as mercaptopurine and azathioprine are constrained to cases that have neglected to react to sulfasalazine and glucocorticoids.

The Anti-Inflammatory Diet for Arthritis Relief

Nourishment and arthritis have an association with one another, and that is why changing your diet is one of the main recommendations a specialist can give an individual with irritation in their joints. Some sustenances can diminish aggravation, and some may decline the irritation. An individual with arthritis ought to pursue the mitigating diet if the person in question needs to get treated. To begin a mitigating diet, one should know which nourishments the person is going to take out in one's diet and which sustenances will be included.

What are the nourishments that you ought to keep away from and dispose of in your diet? When it comes to arthritis, it is continuously exhorted that the individual influenced ought to kill artificial nourishments like shoddy nourishments, those sustenances that have been handled and sustenances with included artificial flavorings and colorings. An individual with arthritis ought to likewise stay away from meats that have abnormal amounts of fats and sustenances that are high in sugar. The reasons why these sorts of nourishments ought to be evaded by individuals with arthritis is that the soaked fats and trans fats found in these sorts of sustenances can intensify one's condition. The individual ought to likewise maintain a strategic distance from potatoes, eggplants, and tomatoes because these are a piece of the nightshade group of plant that contains solanine that can incite the agony. Cutting these sorts of vegetables in individuals with arthritis have not been demonstrated at this point to be successful. However, the individuals who pursued this sort of diet regularly show enhancements with their condition and discover help from torment.

What are the nourishments to be included in your diet if you have arthritis? If you know which sorts of nourishments you ought to take out in your mitigating diet, you should now realize sustenances to add to your diet:

1. Solid fats and Oils: Fish oils are high in Omega-3 unsaturated fats that are fundamental to the wellbeing. This will help decrease the aggravation and keep it from returning. You will likewise get these fats in certain seeds like flaxseed, pumpkin seeds, and sunflower seeds and furthermore in Brazil nuts, almonds, cashew nuts and some more.

2. Products of the soil: You ought to eat more foods grown from the ground if you have arthritis because these have a ton of mineral, nutrients, cell reinforcements and photochemical that are gainful for your arthritis and furthermore to different conditions.

3. Protein: Eating more proteins like fishes and different kinds of seafood and poultry meats will likewise help individuals with arthritis.

4. Beverages: You should require more fluids to keep your joints greased up. Drink more water, natural product juices, tea, vegetable juice with low sodium and non-fat milk.

Treating yourself for arthritis isn't difficult if you know the sort of diet that is proper for your condition and if you realize the sustenances to maintain a strategic distance from with arthritis just as the nourishments that must be eaten.

Elective Cures for Arthritis

Arthritis causes medical issues and incapacities in almost 70 million Americans, or around one in every three grown-ups, and the numbers are just on the ascent. Arthritis symptoms can change from gentle to extreme, now and again notwithstanding prompting handicap. Around 17% of incapacity cases are brought about by arthritis, bringing about colossal expenses for the individual, their families, and the state.

Arthritis isn't a disease; however, a gathering of diseases whose shared factor is irritation, stiffness, restricted development, torment, and devastation of the joints. Three out of 5 arthritis sufferers are younger than 65, so arthritis isn't only a disease of the older.

The most well-known structure is Osteoarthritis, which is otherwise called mileage arthritis". It is regularly thought of as by result of the maturing procedure like silver hair, and wrinkles. Osteoarthritis begins for the most part in the middle age, sometime before the principal symptoms are taken note. The ligament that covers the bone starts to break down, enabling unresolved issues together. Bone spikes and sores are basic advancements. During this degeneration procedure, the muscles, ligaments, and tendons may wind up stressed, causing aggravation and agony. The fundamental issue with Osteoarthritis is torment; aggravation is an issue in the later phases of arthritis. Here and there is no torment, yet the influenced joints free scope of movement and become stiff.

Osteoarthritis shows up in two general structures, essential and auxiliary. Essential Osteoarthritis is the more typical structure, is a moderate and dynamic condition that usually strikes after the age of 45, influencing, for the most part, the weight-bearing joints of the knees and hips, just as the lower back, neck, huge toe and finger joints. It creates by putting inordinate loads on a joint or when a sensible burden is set on a second rate joint. The definite reason is yet to be resolved, even though heredity and weight are hazard factors.

Auxiliary Osteoarthritis shows up ordinarily because of injury or damage to the joint (like football damage or auto collision), uneven metabolic characters (gout or calcium stores, iron over-burden, thyroid disease, or long haul utilization of specific meds), joint contamination, or even medical procedure. It strikes individuals more youthful than 45. Injury gives off an impression of being the principle explanation behind creating Osteoarthritis. The injury could be intense (mishap) or constant (repeating after some time). Interminable damage makes total harm the joint. The beginning usually is felt like a little uneasiness that ends up extreme and crippling after some time. An insecure or free joint given a torn tendon would be a case of this. Dull effect stacking is another type of interminable injury. This includes a dull movement that damages the joint tissue (baseball pitcher, drill administrator, ballet dancer). Dull effect stacking is one of the primary drivers of optional Osteoarthritis, particularly in joints that are as of now experiencing anomalous arrangement or that are utilized in manners that they shouldn't be. Not all-high pressure action harms joint tissues, the more significant part of them can. Osteoarthritis may likewise be the reason due to poor bone arrangement, inappropriately framed joints, or the way you walk.

Osteoarthritis and Rheumatoid arthritis are frequently befuddled because of the comparability in their names. Rheumatoid arthritis is an immune system disease that makes the body's invulnerable framework assault its tissues. It causes shortcoming, exhaustion, fever, frailty, and different issues, including aggravated joints. Rheumatoid arthritis tends to strikes evenly, which means it strikes the two joints (left and right half of the body). It at first strikes between the ages of 25 and 50, versus Osteoarthritis for the most part after

45. RA regularly travels every which way all of a sudden; OA grows step by step more than quite a while. OA starts in a single joint. RA symptoms are redness, warmth, and swelling, in OA, these symptoms are strange in the beginning times. RA influences numerous or most joints like knees, knuckles, wrists, elbows, and shoulders. OA influences joints of the hands, hips, feet, and spine, and just every so often assaults different joints. RA causes a general sentiment of ailment and weakness, just as weight reduction and fever; OA doesn't cause a general sentiment of affliction.

It is the basic agreement that arthritis is hopeless, and must be made to do with agony and mitigating prescription. This treatment plan will cover the symptoms and won't address the hidden causes so that the disease can advance further. Likewise, these medications have genuine reactions. A large number of individuals bite the dust each year from unfavorable symptoms of mitigating, acetaminophen, and steroids.

Solid ligament needs three things; water for oil and sustenance, proteoglycans to draw in and hold the water, and collagen to keep the proteoglycans set up.

There are elective treatment plans accessible to can be of extraordinary assistance to the person living with arthritis.

Sustenance Link to arthritis, nourishment sensitivities, and bigotries could exasperate and cause arthritis. Keeping your body at a perfect weight, and providing your body with every one of the supplements it needs to remake muscle and bone tissue is significant and eating an alkalizing diet that incorporates crisp leafy foods, lean protein, and complex starches, and decreasing sugar and awful fats. Arthritis is a disease of an over an acidic framework. Rehearsing bit control and growing great dietary patterns will enable you to free weight and look after it while feeling much improved and increasingly vigorous. Point of confinement your purine consumption, purines is found in organ meats, anchovies, and sardines. Overabundance purine levels in the blood lead to uric corrosive, which has been connected to Gout and arthritis. Liquor builds likewise increments uric corrosive creation. Admission of refined sugar negatively affects glucose balance, the insusceptible framework, and advances aggravation. The group of nightshade of vegetables, similar to tomatoes, eggplants, potatoes, and peppers is the most well-known offenders to cause a joint condition.

Expanding your water admission can be of extraordinary assistance. Numerous constant wellbeing conditions are brought about by ceaseless drying out. You can kill various issues by only drinking more water.

Supplementations can be of extraordinary advantage if the correct measurements and the right item are utilized. This will decide whether the supplementation will be viable. The three most encouraging enhancements for arthritis endures are Glucosamine, chondroitin, and ASU.

Glucosamine comprises of glucose and the corrosive amino glutamine. It is a significant piece of the mucopolysaccharides, which give structure deep down, ligament, skin, nails, hair, and other body tissue. Glucosamine is a noteworthy structure square of the proteoglycans.

The suggested measurements for Glucosamine HCL it is 1500 mg, or 1884 mg for Glucosamine sulfate once every day or twice separated into two equivalent portions. Glucosamine sulfate is the structure utilized in generally examine. Glucosamine HCL is to some degree like, because Glucosamine sulfate should be balanced out with salt or potassium. This could prompt an undesirable ascent in circulatory strain, depending on how much salt or potassium was included.

Chondroitin works like the regular happening chondroitin in the body's ligament; it shields the old ligament from untimely breakdown and animates the blend of the new ligament.

The prescribed dose for Chondroitin is 800 to 1200 mg once day by day or twice partitioned into two equivalent portions.

Glucosamine and Chondroitin taking together are liked because they work synergistically. They animate blend of new ligament, while all the while controlling the ligament annihilating chemicals, and keeping the chondrocytes sound.

These enhancements are treating the disease on a cellular level, helping the body mend itself while torment drugs veil the symptoms of the disease.

ASU is a characteristic vegetable concentrate produced using Avocado and Soybean oils. Avocado Soybean Unsaponifables has been a solution treatment for osteoarthritis in France since the mid-1990s. ASU differs from Glucosamine and Chondroitin because it is a blend of a wide range of plant substances. ASU originates from the common avocado and soybean oils; the enhancements proportion is one section avocado to 2 sections soybean. The handling of ASU is exceptionally mind-boggling and costly. ASU is significantly more convoluted than making Glucosamine and Chondroitin. There are different dynamic fixings in ASU that need cautious taking care of to be purified and balanced out. A few organizations are selling avocado and soy oils, and not the dynamic ASU fixings. Avocado and Soy oils don't contain similar active parts, in similar amounts, as the profoundly handled, purified, and amassed fixings as in the legitimate items.

Prescribed measurements for ASU is 300 mg once day by day.

When purchasing any enhancement, you need to ensure that it is of good quality. One approach to guarantee this is to buy items that cling to Good Manufacturing Protocols. The crate ought to have GMP stepped on it. The item could be the second rate regardless of whether the mark expresses that it is "research center tried." This could allude to the crude material, which is extremely uncertain, and numerous things can occur during the time spent enhancing. Just testing of the finished result is a satisfactory type of guaranteeing exact readings. Taking second rate items, ones that don't utilize quality fixings or items that are not fabricated with the best possible controls is an exercise in futility and cash. Shockingly this is the situation with most items available today.

Chondroitin is costlier to make than Glucosamine. Thus organizations are more enthusiasm for benefit than quality may attempt to hold back on chondroitin by giving not accurately is recorded on the mark; utilizing doses lower than those bolstered by research; substituting less expensive, less dynamic, or dormant substances; getting chondroitin from organizations that don't pursue the strictest quality gauges in handling.

Every one of the three items is generally safe. Glucosamine is alright for diabetics; it conveys the equivalent of sugar as a grape. Most of the Glucosamine is fabricated from the shells of lobsters, shrimp, and crab. The meat protein that causes the unfavorably susceptible response isn't found in the shell. Individuals with shellfish hypersensitivity ought to be cautious and ask their PCP or take Regenasure, the veggie lover structure. There are no reports on unfriendly responses. There is no proof to help the risk contracting frantic dairy animals' disease from Chondroitin. The microscopic organisms would be murdered during preparing.

Know about items that guarantee to be durable, time-discharged, or control conveyance. Glucosamine, Chondroitin, and ASU are dependable themselves. Additionally, for the best outcomes, you need them to be discharged as fast as could be allowed.

Twofold and triple quality items show that you have to take fewer tablets to accomplish similar outcomes. This necessarily implies bigger tablets, which is anything but a smart thought for someone that has an issue gulping.

Fluid enhancements are typically not as steady as powders or containers. There is no proof that fluid ingests superior to containers, in this specific case. It is conceivable that retention is lower in fluid items. Stomach corrosive is significant for appropriate retention of glucosamine. The liquid items could weaken the corrosive, meddling with retention. There is additionally an issue with poor taste, and drinking more water to veil it, again weakening the item.

Be careful of the word complex in Glucosamine/Chondroitin items. It, for the most part, implies that different substances have been included, similar to manganese or

Nutrient C. It could likewise imply that the item was weakened with N-acetyl glucosamine. This could prompt a decreased adequacy of the intensity. Chondroitin complex, as a rule, implies that mediocre items are utilized, like MSM, hydrolyzed collagen, chicken ligament, and related substances that are not Chondroitin. This decreases cost and brings more benefit to the maker; however, harms the shopper by giving them a faulty item.

Stay away from topical structures. Glucosamine and Chondroitin are pointless if connected topically.

Use alert if there is an unconditional promise. Most makers profit with delivery alone.

Be wary if something professes to be superior to Glucosamine and Chondroitin, except for ASU, there is nothing to help this case scientifically.

Stay away from store brands. The FDA does not carefully direct dietary enhancements. There is nothing of the sort as a "nonexclusive" supplement - there are just tremendous or poor enhancements. You are most likely not getting the dynamic fixings you need in a store brand.

Item quality stays as the most significant hindrance in utilizing glucosamine/chondroitin and ASU supplements. When purchasing these items make a point to purchase from an organization that pursues great assembling rehearses; buy items that have likewise been tried and suggested by autonomous research facilities.

Different enhancements that are gainful incorporate Vitamin C, Vitamin B 6, Vitamin E, Magnesium, Omega 3s, Selenium, Calcium, and Boron.

Exercise and Rest: You need to move to remain sound. Exercise assists with course, venous and lymph return, squander disposal, conditions your muscles and inner organs, and your joints. The ligament in your joints has no blood supply and relies upon moving them to support them and expel squander items. Weight-bearing activity keeps your bones solid, and to avoid Osteoporosis. Yoga and extending improve adaptability and stretch muscles. Cardio activities promote the course and waste disposal. Exercise in itself discharges feel-great hormones in the body and is gainful for gloom and mental prosperity.

It is critical to get legitimate rest around evening time, so the body gets an opportunity to energize itself. Not allowing your body to restore will leave you feeling unfilled and drained.

Reflection and Relaxation: There is a connection between stress and incessant wellbeing conditions. The more you center around something, the higher it will turn into. If you are in steady torment, you will concentrate on it, and it will end up being your perspective. This is justifiable. However, it will just bring you more torment. Learning unwinding strategies like contemplation, biofeedback, the perception among others, will support you discharge negative pressure, and feel much improved.

Needle therapy and Chinese Medicine: see wellbeing as nonattendance of disease, yet as an amicable condition of body, brain, and soul. In Chinese drug, your wellbeing is dictated by your capacity to adjust your yin and yang, the two contradicting powers that makeup everything known to man. The indispensable vitality of the body or qi is hindered when yin and yang are out of parity, bringing about torment and disease. Setting up equalization and agreement in the body will bring about wellbeing.

Ayurvedic: Ayurveda signifies "information of life." It speaks to a whole way of thinking of life and living. The customer is guided on the most proficient method to create self-information and figure out how to address awkward nature to acquire wellbeing. The customer will take a shot at reinforcing their prana (life power) by blending their dosha or established sort. The medicines include diet and sustenance, herbs, yoga works out, reflection, back rub, and breathing activities.

Chiropractic and Osteopathy: the two modalities expect to bring the body once more into the arrangement by changing the bones of the body. The sensory system is brought once again into legitimate working request by reestablishing appropriate equalization to the spinal segment and joints, permitting nerve driving forces to travel unreservedly from the cerebrum through the spinal section to all body parts. Blocked blood and nerve stream brings about agony and disease, if not adjusted.

Herbs: Herb medication and fragrance based treatment use plants, herbs, and other regular substances to invigorate the body to come back to the condition of wellbeing. Even though herbs are prescriptions, they will, in general, be a lot more secure than substance drugs for some reasons; they are less intense, increasingly conspicuous to the body, and normally utilized in mixes and potencies that limit adverse reactions.

Homeopathy: depends on the idea that "Preferences fix loves." This implies prescription ought not to be utilized to balance symptoms, however, to invigorate the body's very own recuperating powers.

Back rub and Bodywork: are exceptionally gainful for people with arthritis. Back massage will improve the course, lymph stream, squander disposal, give unwinding to sore muscles and joints, and diminish pressure and tension levels in the body.

What conditions can anti-inflammatory diet help?

Doctors, dietitians, and naturopaths suggest mitigating diets as a complementary therapy for many conditions that are exacerbated by constant aggravation.

An anti-inflammatory diet can help many conditions, including:

- Rheumatoid joint inflammation
- Psoriasis
- Asthma
- Eosinophilic esophagitis
- Crohn's illness
- Colitis
- Fiery entrail illness
- Diabetes
- Weight
- Metabolic disorder
- Coronary illness
- Lupus
- Hashimoto's illness

Moreover, eating an anti-inflammatory diet can help reduce the danger of specific malignant growths, including colorectal disease.

Best Foods to eat

Significant decisions for a person following a mitigating diet incorporate the accompanying:

Dim verdant greens, including kale and spinach

Blueberries, blackberries, and fruits

Dim red grapes

Sustenance thick vegetables, for example, broccoli and cauliflower

Beans and lentils

Green tea

Red wine, with some restraint

Avocado and coconut

Olives

Additional virgin olive oil

Pecans, pistachios, pine nuts, and almonds

Cold-water fish, including salmon and sardines

Turmeric and cinnamon

Dim chocolate

Flavors and herbs

Sustenances to stay away from

The basic sustenances that people following the anti-inflammatory diet ought to stay away from include:

Handled meats

Sugary beverages

Trans fats, found in broiled nourishments

White bread

White pasta

Gluten

Soybean oil and vegetable oil

Handled nibble nourishments, for example, chips and saltines

Pastries, for example, treats, sweets, and frozen yogurt

Overabundance liquor

Such a large number of carbohydrates

Conclusion

A few people find that nourishments in the nightshades family, for example, tomatoes, eggplants, peppers, and potatoes, can trigger flares in some incendiary maladies. There is limited evidence of this. However, a person can take a stab at cutting nightshades from the diet for 2–3 weeks to check whether their manifestations improve.

There is some evidence that recommends a high-carbohydrate diet, notwithstanding when the carbs are refreshing, may advance aggravation. Along these lines, many people on a mitigating diet choose to reduce their carbohydrate consumption.

Can a vegetarian diet reduce irritation?

People considering a mitigating diet may likewise need to consider wiping out meat for vegetarian protein sources or greasy fish.

Research recommends that people following a vegetarian diet have larger amounts of plasma AA, a marker of generally speaking wellbeing that is related to lower levels of irritation and coronary illness.

An examination found that eating creature items expanded the danger of fundamental irritation, while another investigation proposes that reduced aggravation is one of the critical advantages of a veggie lover diet.

anti-inflammatory diet tips

Calming diets might be a significant change for people who will, in general, eat various types of sustenance.

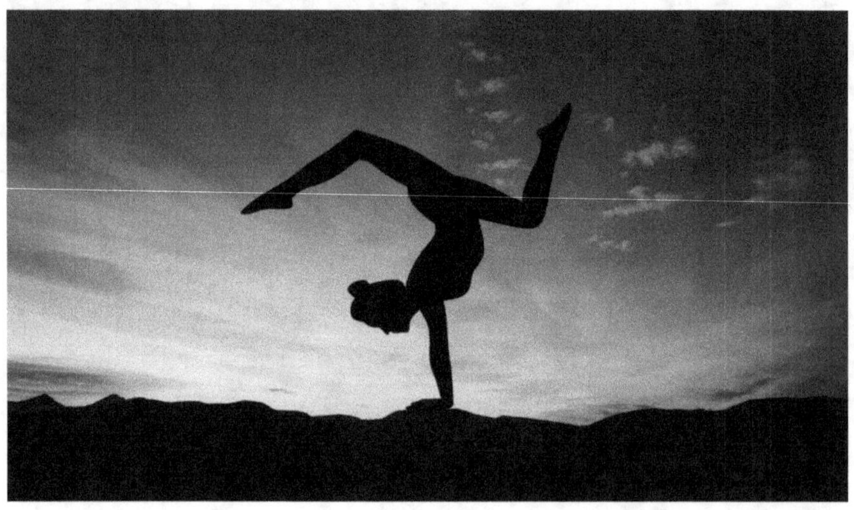